STRUGGLES AND ADVANTAGES OF THE ADVENTIST HEALTH MESSAGE

Pr. Ebenezer Ankomah
LOVE, OBEY AND LIVE MINISTRY
SEPTEMBER, 2020

DEDICATION

This book is dedicated to the almighty God, my lovely wife and daughter, my immediate family, friends and God's people everywhere who desire to know and obey a "thus saith the Lord." Also to all lecturers and students of the Adventist University of Africa (AUA), Kenya.

TABLE OF CONTENTS

CHAPTER 1

INTRODUCTION

Seventh-day Adventists are known to be Christians who "proclaim the everlasting gospel embraced in the three angels' messages [Revelation 14:6–12]."[1] The Adventist Health Message (AHM) is seen to be "connected with the third angel's message, and is to work efficiently as the right arm, for the defense of the body of truth."[2] As such, Adventist are known also for the proclamation of the Health Message to promote the quality of lives of individuals in both the church and the society at large. Joyce Hopp and Neish records that "the Seventh-day

---

[1]The Seventh-day Adventist Church has as its mission statement "to call all people to become disciples of Jesus Christ, to proclaim the everlasting gospel embraced in the three angels' messages [Revelation 14:6–12], and to prepare the world for Christ's soon return." accessed September 2, 2018, https://www.adventist.org/en/information/official-statements/statements/article/go/-/mission-statement-of-the-seventh-day-adventist-church/.

[2]Ellen G. White, *Review and Herald, June 20, 1899,* Complete Published Ellen G. White Writings, Comprehensive Research Edition [CD ROM] (Silver Spring, MD: Ellen G. White Estate, 2012), par. 10.

Adventist health message has been an integral part of church beliefs and practice since the denomination's beginnings as an organized entity."[3]

The Health Message, currently referred to as the Adventist Health Message (AHM) according to Galvez[4] refers to the statements, declarations, and orientations on health, disease and healing written by E. G. White, a pioneer of the Seventh-day Adventist Church.[5]

The AHM has been through many struggles yet it has been so beneficial to its adherents. The advantages in the quality of life and longevity of the Adventist population over the rest of the population in the United States of America and Europe have been proven by research.[6]

This book seeks to address the struggles and advantages of the Adventist Health Message (AHM). The research would first look at the origin and content of the

---

[3]Joyce W. Hopp and Christine Neish,"A Study of the Seventh-day Adventist Health Message," *The Journal of Adventist Education*, December 2009/January 2010, 36.

[4]Cesar Augusto Galvez "A Wholeness Approach for the Adventist Health Message," *ResearchGate*, November 2016, 114.

[5]Ibid., 115.

[6]G. E. Fraser, *Diet, Life Expectancy, and Chronic Diseases: Studies of Seventh Day Adventist and other Vegetarian*, (New York, NY: Oxford University, 2003).

Adventist Health Message (AHM) by exploring various documents of the Seventh-day Adventist Church. Having done that, it will then proceed to the struggles and the advantages of the AHM.

CHAPTER 2

ORIGIN OF THE ADVENTIST HEALTH MESSAGE

It is believed that the AHM was communicated by God through Ellen G. White in vision to the Church and the world at large. Ellen White writes, "It was at the house of Bro. A. Hilliard, at Otsego, Mich., June 6, 1863, that the great subject of Health Reform was opened before me in vision."[7] Thus the AHM dates back to the prophetic visions of E. G. White on June 6, 1863.

This vision occurred at a prayer and song service held at the beginning of the Sabbath. An eye-witness to this vision has written: "Sister White was asked to lead in prayer at family worship. She did so in a most wonderful manner. Elder White was kneeling a short distance from her. While praying, she moved over to him, and laying her hand on his shoulder continued praying for him until she

---

[7] Ellen G. White, *Review and Herald, October 8, 1867,* Complete Published Ellen G. White Writings, Comprehensive Research Edition [CD ROM] (Silver Spring, MD: Ellen G. White Estate, 2012), par. 3.

was taken off in vision. She was in vision about forty-five minutes. It was at this time she was given instruction upon the health question which soon after became such a matter of interest to our people."[8]

E. G. White wrote about her experience in the vision of June 6, 1863: "I saw that it was a sacred duty to attend to our health, and arouse others to their duty, and yet not take the burden of their case upon us." She continued that "we have a duty to speak, to come out against intemperance of every kind--intemperance in working, in eating, in drinking, and in drugging--and then point them to God's great medicine, water, pure soft water, for diseases, for health, for cleanliness, and for a luxury."[9] D. E. Robbinson asserts that the document containing this statement is still preserved in the original handwriting.[10]

---

[8]Mrs. Martha D. Amadon, Ellen G. White Publications, Document File No. 105, accessed September 12, 2018, https://m.egwwritings.org/en/book/660.1395.

[9]Ellen G. White, *Manuscript Releases, vol. 5,* Complete Published Ellen G. White Writings, Comprehensive Research Edition [CD ROM] (Silver Spring, MD: Ellen G. White Estate, 2012), 105.3.

[10]D. E. Robbinson, *The Story of our Health Message,* 3rd ed. (Nashville TN: Southern Pub. Ass., 1965), 77.

CHAPTER 3

CONTENT OF THE ADVENTIST HEALTH MESSAGE

E. G. White clearly stated in her writings that "failure to care for the living machinery is an insult to the Creator." In view of this, God has "divinely appointed rules which if observed will keep human beings from disease and premature death."[11]

The AHM is based on what E. G. White saw in her 1863 vision. In this vision, she was shown some 33 core health principles which has become the clear, sensible practical outline of the lifestyle of Seventh-day Adventists.[12]

These core principles are: "1. Those who do not control their appetite in eating are guilty of intemperance. 2. Swine's flesh is not to be eaten under any circumstance.

---

[11]Ellen G. White, *Counsels on Diet and Foods,* Complete Published Ellen G. White Writings, Comprehensive Research Edition [CD ROM] (Silver Spring, MD: Ellen G. White Estate, 2012), 16.4.

[12]Herbert E. Douglass, *Messenger of the Lord,* 3rd ed. (Oakland CA: Pacific Press, 1998), 283, 284.

3. Tobacco in any form is a slow poison. 4. Strict cleanliness of the body and home premises is important. 5. Tea and coffee, similar to tobacco, are slow poisons. 6. Rich cake, pies, and puddings are injurious. 7. Eating between meals injures the stomach and digestive process. 8. Adequate time must be allowed between meals, giving the stomach time to rest. 9. If a third meal is taken, it should be light and several hours before bedtime. 10. People used to meat, gravies, and pastries do not immediately relish a plain, wholesome diet. 11. Gluttonous appetite contributes to indulgence of corrupt passions. 12. Turning to a plain, nutritious diet may overcome the physical damage caused by a wrong diet. 13. Reforms in eating will save expense and labor. 14. Children eating flesh meat and spicy foods have strong tendencies toward sexual indulgences. 15. Poisonous drugs used as medical prescriptions kill more people than all other causes of death combined. 16. Pure water should be used freely in maintaining health and curing illnesses. 17. Nature alone has curative powers. 18. Common medicines, such as strychnine, opium, calomel, mercury, and quinine, are poisons. 19. Parents transmit their weaknesses to their children; prenatal influences are enormous. 20. Obeying the laws of health will prevent many illnesses. 21. God is too often blamed for deaths

caused by violation of nature's laws. 22. Light and pure air are required, especially in the sleeping quarters. 23. Bathing, even a sponge bath, will be beneficial on rising in the morning. 24. God will not work healing miracles for those who continually violate the laws of health. 25. Many invalids have no physical cause for their illness; they have a diseased imagination. 26. Cheerful, physical labor will help to create a healthy, cheerful disposition. 27. Willpower has much to do with resisting disease and soothing nerves. 28. Outdoor exercise is very important to health of mind and body. 29. Overwork breaks down both mind and body; routine daily rest is necessary. 30. Many die of disease caused wholly by eating flesh food. 31. Caring for health is a spiritual matter, reflecting a person's commitment to God. 32. A healthy mind and body directly affects one's morals and one's ability to discern truth. 33. All God's promises are given on condition of obedience."[13]

E. G. White in her book, *The Ministry of Healing* often amplified these core principles. The AHM is captured in one of her popular statements: "Pure air, sunlight, abstemiousness, rest, exercise, proper diet, the use of water,

---

[13] Herbert E. Douglass, *Messenger of the Lord,* 3rd ed. (Oakland CA: Pacific Press, 1998), 283, 284.

trust in divine power--these are the true remedies."[14]
Throughout her writings, E. G. White called for a balanced
approach to health reforms by avoiding various extremes.

[14]Ellen G. White, *The Ministry of Healing*, Complete
Published Ellen G. White Writings, Comprehensive Research Edition
[CD ROM] (Silver Spring, MD: Ellen G. White Estate, 2012), 127.2.

CHAPTER 4

STRUGGLES OF THE ADVENTIST HEALTH MESSAGE

The AHM produces a healthy lifestyle which provides "the best condition for the highest service to God and man."[15] Nevertheless, it has gone through struggles throughout the ages.

E. G. White herself did not get it easy. She went through various struggles when she received the health message. She recounts, "I suffered keen hunger, I was a great meat eater. But when faint, I placed my arms across my stomach, and said: 'I will not taste a morsel. I will eat simple food, or I will not eat at all.' . . . When I made these changes I had a special battle to fight."[16] The good news is that she was victorious over her struggles with the truth of

---

[15]Ibid., 319.1

[16]Ellen G. White, *Testimonies for the Church*, vol. 2, Complete Published Ellen G. White Writings, Comprehensive Research Edition [CD ROM] (Silver Spring, MD: Ellen G. White Estate, 2012), 371.2.

health reform. E. G. White later reported that "I have left [off] the use of meat."[17] Again, she wrote to her son, "We have in diet been strict to follow the light the Lord has given us."[18]

Aside the struggles of E. G. White herself, the AHM has been through various struggles in the hands of its recipients. Below are some of them.

Making the health message a criterion for salvation is one of the major struggles of the AHM. The experience of Limoni Manu is a typical example of how misunderstanding of the health message can be very dangerous. Manu writes "twenty years ago it seemed crystal clear to me: Nonvegetarian Adventists will not enter heaven. And I shared my faith with everyone who would lend me an ear."[19] His argument was based on E. G. White's statement: "among those who are waiting for the

---

[17]Ellen G. White, *Spiritual Gift vol. 4A*, Complete Published Ellen G. White Writings, Comprehensive Research Edition [CD ROM] (Silver Spring, MD: Ellen G. White Estate, 2012), 153.3

[18] Ellen G. White, *Manuscript Releases vol. 14*, Complete Published Ellen G. White Writings, Comprehensive Research Edition [CD ROM] (Silver Spring, MD: Ellen G. White Estate, 2012), 312.2.

[19]Limoni Manu, "Nonvegetarian Will Not Enter Heaven? Guidelines for Interpreting Ellen White on the Topic of Health" *Adventist Review,* 2005, accessed September 2, 2018, http://archives.adventistreview.org/2005-1538/story2.html.

coming of the Lord, meat eating will eventually be done away; flesh will cease to form a part of their diet. We should ever keep this end in view, and endeavor to work steadily toward it."[20] Most people like Manu struggle with eisegesis and misconstrue the health message as a measuring rod for salvation.

Another struggle of the AHM is extremes in health reform. Many have taken health reform to the various extremes. E. G. White asserts that "not all who profess to believe in dietetic reform are really reformers. With many persons the reform consists merely in discarding certain unwholesome foods."[21] Many people who do not understand health principles go to the extreme of loading their tables with harmful dainties. Another class adopt an impoverished diet whiles others think that "there need be little care in the selection or the preparation of food," restricting "themselves to a very meagre diet, not having sufficient variety to supply the needs of the system."[22] She

---

[20]Ellen G. White, *Counsels on Diet and Foods,* Complete Published Ellen G. White Writings, Comprehensive Research Edition [CD ROM] (Silver Spring, MD: Ellen G. White Estate, 2012), 380.4.

[21]Ellen G. White, *The Ministry of Healing*, Complete Published Ellen G. White Writings, Comprehensive Research Edition [CD ROM] (Silver Spring, MD: Ellen G. White Estate, 2012), 318.1.

[22]Ibid., 318, 319.

states that "health reform becomes health deform, a health destroyer, when it is carried to extremes."[23]

Irrational reform is also another struggle of the AHM. There is the need for applying common sense in dietary reforms when it comes to practice in real life situation. Broad and deep study of the subject is required by all. Unfortunately, many have embarked and have urged others to embark on health reform without rationally considering the matter. This attitude has caused many to shun the AHM. E. G. White's counsel is beneficial here: "One person cannot be a standard for everybody else. What we want is a little sprinkling of good common sense."[24]

The last of the struggles I would like to talk about is insensitive reforms. Sensitive factors like changes in climate, age, the impact of the economy, the availability of fruits and vegetables and other things help to decide the best food item to choose in different environments. Unfortunately, many embark on health reform without paying attention to these sensitive factors. This is very

---

[23]Ellen G. White, *Counsels on Diet and Foods,* Complete Published Ellen G. White Writings, Comprehensive Research Edition [CD ROM] (Silver Spring, MD: Ellen G. White Estate, 2012), 202.4.

[24]Ellen G. White, *Sermons and Talks* Complete Published Ellen G. White Writings, Comprehensive Research Edition [CD ROM] (Silver Spring, MD: Ellen G. White Estate, 2012), 12.2.

dangerous. While health reform is a necessity, it is very important to consider to the various sensitive factors.

CHAPTER 5

ADVANTAGES OF THE ADVENTIST HEALTH
MESSAGE

The AHM has been of tremendous Advantage to humanity since the 1860s. It has been the pledge of God Himself "to keep this living machinery in healthful action if the human agent will obey his laws, and co-operate with him."[25] Those who have lived in obedience to the AHM have enjoyed the blessings of God in keeping them healthy and joyful. Below are some of the advantages accrued from obeying the AHM.

1. Improved health and long life: Among Adventists who accepted the health reform message in the 1860s, R. M. Kilgore, a longtime evangelist-administrator writes "As they advanced, they felt their diseases, aches, and pains leaving them, and in return buoyancy of spirit,

---

[25]Ellen G. White, *Healthful Living,* Complete Published Ellen G. White Writings, Comprehensive Research Edition [CD ROM] (Silver Spring, MD: Ellen G. White Estate, 2012), 22.5.

and glow of health, the greatest earthly blessings."[26] It has been proven by research that Adventists in general live longer and healthier than the rest of the human population who live close to them. For instance, "in the Netherlands those that joined the Adventist church by 27 years of age lived longer than non-Adventists by 8.9 years for women and 3.6 years for men. For lifetime Adventists in Norway life expectancy was 5.2 years longer for Adventists compared to non-Adventists. In early studies California Adventist females lived on average 6.2 years longer than non-Adventists and males lived 3.7 years longer. Later studies of California Adventists revealed even greater differences, with Adventist women and men living on average 7.3 and 4.4 years longer than non-Adventists, respectively. Vegetarian California Adventists lived 2.5 longer for females and 1.7 for males compared to non-vegetarian California Adventists."[27]

2. Better Cure of Diseases: It is known from medical science that "from the homely aspirin to the most

---

[26]Herbert E. Douglass, Messenger of the Lord, 3rd Ed. (Oakland CA: Pacific Press, 1998), 301.

[27]Wayne S. Dysinger, "The Adventist Advantage," accessed September 2, 2018, http://aplaceofhealing.info/health-smart-online/31-section-xii-philosophy-of-health-and-healing-/185-chapter-4-the-adventist-advantage.html.

sophisticated prescription medicine on the market, all drugs come with side effects."[28] The administration of drugs into the body may seem to be of beneficial effect when a change takes place for a time. However, the disease is not cured. Mrs. White asserts that "drugs never cure disease. They only change its form and location. Nature alone is the effectual restorer."[29] Again she wrote: "more deaths have been caused by drug-taking than from all other causes combined."[30] The AHM promotes the use of natural remedies to cure diseases instead of using drugs. Natural remedies offer a better cure with no adverse effect on the system.

3. Self-Discipline: It is an established fact that "Self-discipline is required to achieve optimal health when breaking a habit (e.g., smoking) or rebalancing health

---

[28]Melinda Ratini, "Drug Side Effects Explained," accessed September 11, 2018, https://www.webmd.com/a-to-z-guides/drug-side-effects-explained#1.

[29]Ellen G. White, *Review and Herald, September 5, 1899,* Complete Published Ellen G. White Writings, Comprehensive Research Edition [CD ROM] (Silver Spring, MD: Ellen G. White Estate, 2012), par. 4.

[30]Ibid., par. 1.

issues caused by excess."[31] The Adventist health message advocates temperance in all things. It is impossible to obey the AHM without self-discipline. Those who are able to control the appetite are better able to practice self-control in other areas of their lives. Thus, the Adventist health message leads to self-discipline, a necessity to overcome temptation.

4. Reduced risk of lifestyle diseases: Diseases like diabetes, cancers, stroke, heart disease and other cardiovascular diseases are greatly altered by an individual's lifestyle, especially dietary habits and smoking of cigarette. Since the AHM promotes exercise, not drinking alcohol, not smoking, the consumption of healthy foods involving more plant-based diet and less or even total avoidance of meat, fish and other dairy products, there is a reduced risk of lifestyle diseases among Adventists around the globe. Research has proven that deaths of Adventists from diseases of the heart were less than one-third that of non-Adventists in California[32] and that changes in diet

---

[31] Adventist HealthCare, "Self-Discipline," accessed https://blog.adventisthealthcare.com/2013/01/22/the-importance-of-self-discipline/.

[32] Phillips R. L., Kuzma J. W., Beeson W. L., and Lotz T., "Influence of Selection versus Lifestyle on Risk of Fatal Cancer and Cardiovascular Disease Among Seventh-day Adventists," *American Journal of Epidemiology* 112(2) (1980): 296-314.

potentially reduces cancer deaths in the United States by 35%.[33]

5. Effectiveness in labour: Productivity in any line of work is highly dependent on the health of people involved. Healthy people are more productive. This is because healthy people use every faculty of the human machinery during labour. In a research to determine "practical estimates of the costs of productivity loss related to health," it was concluded that "health conditions and lifestyle risk factors are associated with workplace productivity loss." If carefully followed, the AHM leads to health of the entire human being which enables the human machinery to function to its optimum level. This helps to increase productivity in any line of work.

---

[33]Richard Doll and Richard Peto, "The causes of cancer: Quantitative Estimates of Avoidable Risks of Cancer in the United States Today," *Journal of the National Cancer Institute*, Volume 66, Issue 6, 1 June 1981, Pages 1192–1308, accessed September 12, 2018, https://doi.org/10.1093/jnci/66.6.1192.

CHAPTER 6
SUMMARY AND CONCLUSION

The AHM has been clearly presented in this book. It was observed that the AHM originated with the vision of E. G. White at Otsego, Michigan on June 6, 1863. The AHM emphasized that care of health is a religious duty and that diseases are caused by violation of health laws. It teaches temperance in all things, promotes vegetarianism and the use of natural remedies in healing. Also, personal hygiene and health education are required to keep the human machinery in a healthful condition.

Various struggles of the AHM were presented. Aside E. G. White's personal struggle with the health reform message, making the health message a criterion for salvation, extremes in health reform, irrational reforms and insensitive reforms were the noted struggles of the AHM.

Despite the struggles of AHM, the AHM have some advantages. It has the advantages of improved health and long life, better cure of diseases, reduced risk of lifestyle diseases and self-discipline which leads to effectiveness in labour that increases productivity.

The AHM is a blessing to the Church and the world at large. It is therefore important that we try as much as possible to put the AHM into practice for our own good. We must do so recognizing that "diet reform should be progressive."[34] E. G. White stated that "we do not mark out any precise line to be followed in diet"[35] and "I make myself a criterion for no one else"[36] neither should anyone make himself a criterion for others. Let all with a clear understanding of the AHM use common sense in applying it for a healthy life.

---

[34]Ellen G. White, *The Ministry of Healing*, Complete Published Ellen G. White Writings, Comprehensive Research Edition [CD ROM] (Silver Spring, MD: Ellen G. White Estate, 2012), 320.2.

[35]Ellen G. White, *Testimonies for the Church*, vol. 9, Complete Published Ellen G. White Writings, Comprehensive Research Edition [CD ROM] (Silver Spring, MD: Ellen G. White Estate, 2012), 159.2.

[36]Ellen G. White, *Counsels on Diet and Foods,* Complete Published Ellen G. White Writings, Comprehensive Research Edition [CD ROM] (Silver Spring, MD: Ellen G. White Estate, 2012), 493.5.

BIBLIOGRAPHY

Doll, Richard., and Richard Peto, "The causes of cancer:
Quantitative Estimates of Avoidable Risks of Cancer in
the United States Today." *Journal of the National
Cancer Institute*, Volume 66, Issue 6, 1 June 1981,
Pages 1192–1308. Accessed September 12, 2018,
https://doi.org/10.1093/jnci/66.6.1192.

Douglass, Herbert E. *Messenger of the Lord.* 3rd ed. Oakland
CA: Pacific Press, 1998.

Dysinger, Wayne S. "The Adventist Advantage." Accessed
September 2, 2018, http://aplaceofhealing.info/health-
smart-online/31-section-xii-philosophy-of-health-and-
healing-/185-chapter-4-the-adventist-advantage.html.

Fraser, G. E. *Diet, Life Expectancy, and Chronic Diseases:
Studies of Seventh Day Adventist and other Vegetarian.*
New York, NY: Oxford University, 2003.

Galvez, Cesar Augusto. "A Wholeness Approach for the
Adventist Health Message," *ResearchGate*, November
2016, 114.

Hopp, Joyce W., and Christine Neish, "A Study of the Seventh-
day Adventist Health Message." *The Journal of
Adventist Education*, December 2009/January 2010.

Manu, Limoni. "Nonvegetarian Will Not Enter Heaven?
Guidelines for Interpreting Ellen White on the Topic of
Health." *Adventist Review,* 2005. Accessed September 2,
2018, http://archives.adventistreview.org/2005-
1538/story2.html.

Phillips R. L., Kuzma JW, Beeson WL, and Lotz T, "Influence
     of Selection versus Lifestyle on Risk of Fatal Cancer
     and Cardiovascular Disease Among Seventh-day
     Adventists." *American Journal of Epidemiology* 112(2)
     (1980): 296-314.

Ratini, Melinda "Drug Side Effects Explained." Accessed
     September 11, 2018, https://www.webmd.com/a-to-z-
     guides/drug-side-effects-explained#1.

Robbinson, D. E. *The Story of our Health Message.* 3rd ed.
     Nashville TN: Southern Pub. Ass., 1965.

White, Ellen G. *Counsels on Diet and Foods.* Complete
     Published Ellen G. White Writings, Comprehensive
     Research Edition [CD ROM]. Silver Spring, MD: Ellen
     G. White Estate, 2012.

White, Ellen G. *Manuscript Releases, vol. 5.* Complete
     Published Ellen G. White Writings, Comprehensive
     Research Edition [CD ROM]. Silver Spring, MD: Ellen
     G. White Estate, 2012.

White, Ellen G. *Manuscript Releases vol. 14.* Complete
     Published Ellen G. White Writings, Comprehensive
     Research Edition [CD ROM]. Silver Spring, MD: Ellen
     G. White Estate, 2012.

White, Ellen G. *Review and Herald.* Complete Published Ellen
     G. White Writings, Comprehensive Research Edition
     [CD ROM]. Silver Spring, MD: Ellen G. White Estate,
     2012.

White, Ellen G. *Spiritual Gift vol. 4A.* Complete Published Ellen
     G. White Writings, Comprehensive Research Edition
     [CD ROM]. Silver Spring, MD: Ellen G. White Estate,
     2012.

White, Ellen G. *Testimonies for the Church*, vol. 2. Complete
     Published Ellen G. White Writings, Comprehensive
     Research Edition [CD ROM]. Silver Spring, MD: Ellen
     G. White Estate, 2012.

White, Ellen G. *Testimonies for the Church*, vol. 9. Complete
     Published Ellen G. White Writings, Comprehensive
     Research Edition [CD ROM]. Silver Spring, MD: Ellen
     G. White Estate, 2012.

White, Ellen G. *The Ministry of Healing*. Complete Published
     Ellen G. White Writings, Comprehensive Research
     Edition [CD ROM]. Silver Spring, MD: Ellen G. White
     Estate, 2012.

White, Ellen G. *Sermons and Talks*. Complete Published Ellen
     G. White Writings, Comprehensive Research Edition
     [CD ROM]. Silver Spring, MD: Ellen G. White Estate,
     2012.

White, Ellen G. *Healthful Living*. Complete Published Ellen G.
     White Writings, Comprehensive Research Edition [CD
     ROM]. Silver Spring, MD: Ellen G. White Estate, 2012.

www.ingramcontent.com/pod-product-compliance
Lightning Source LLC
Chambersburg PA
CBHW070748240726
48654CB00010B/1205